ELIZABETH R. SKOGLUND

I'LL BE BETTER IN THE MORNING

ONE PERSON'S JOURNEY WITH CHRONIC FATIGUE SYNDROME

Table of Contents

For my parents who always understood and for all
the physicians who tried and helped

For Elvio Lingua, M.D., who gave it a name

"The so-called life not worth living does not exist."

"To believe in God is to see that life has meaning."

– Viktor Frankl

"I'm here because He has me here."

– Elizabeth R. Skoglund

Acknowledgments

Unlike any other book I've written, *I'll Be Better in the Morning* emerged from the solitude of a medical disorder which deeply and at first anonymously changed the course and quality of my own life. To share it publicly will hopefully help others who suffer silently with a disease whose name is yet either unknown to them or simply known without knowledge of ways to cope with it.

In order to share this with others I am grateful to Lance Wilcox for his editorial skills and for his technological abilities in producing the actual book itself. Once again, John Whorrall Jr. has produced a cover which captures in one glance the totality of what is being said. My thanks go to Rayne Wilcox and Elizabeth Wilcox for their help in practical areas, their prayer support, Rayne's office skills and Elizabeth's insightful summary on the back cover. My deep gratitude goes to Peter-Brian Andersson, M.D., Ph.D., noted neurologist and author, for his helpful critique as I finished the book and for his supportive endorsement on the back cover. Because writing this book has been uniquely solitary and, on an emotional level, difficult to write, I have been grateful for the prayers of so many who are not named here.

"I'll Be Better in the Morning"

Just beyond the Point Pinos Lighthouse in Pacific Grove, adjoining Monterey, California, a large rock jutted out into the ocean. It was my place on those summers when our family spent our vacation in and around Carmel-by-the-Sea. With its flat, smooth surface, my rock, as I called it, provided a comfortable place to think.

I was in my teens and had discovered some of the great Christians of the past, like Hudson Taylor, Amy Carmichael and others. I was challenged by their lives and by certain teachers from the Christian school I attended. Amy Carmichael's words that nothing matters but that which is eternal reverberated in my mind and I spent long periods stretched out on that rock, watching the ocean around me, while I begged God to show me His path for my life.

As the waves splashed gently against my rock I had my own requests for the future: starting a school/orphanage in China. Between reading *Hudson Taylor's Spiritual Secrets*, hearing stories from my aunt, Ruth Benson, who had been a missionary in China, and several unforgettable encounters with Gladys Aylward and her story of her remarkable work in China, China was my life goal. It was a desire which continued through college, although at that point becoming a physician was added to the list. I sought God but I also knew what I wanted the answer to be: China!

God answered my prayer. First He said "wait." And then a decisive "No." Neither China nor medicine were His calling for me. All of that came crashing down on me through CFIDS. In that sense God used CFIDS, one of the worst things that ever happened to me, to do one of the most important things which ever happened to me: He showed me His will for my life. That process came to a peak when I was 21, just after graduation from college.

It was a bright spring day. As I sat on the grassy knoll adjacent to Royce Hall at UCLA, life had technically never been better. I had graduated early with my BA degree in January and was now at the start of graduate school. I was dating a wonderful man, and I planned to begin teaching high school in the fall while I continued part time as a student. Everything looked bright, and yet a dark cloud was slowly rolling in over me. I was tired, not just your average just graduated tired, not that good tired after a hard day's work, but big-time-serious, can't-go-on tired.

Just a week earlier I had taken an exam in a literature class, taught by a professor for whom I had worked as an undergraduate. He knew me well. As I looked at the first question, my mind blurred. I simply couldn't understand what he was asking. When I asked him to explain the question, he looked at me quizzically and said, "Are you okay?" Embarrassed, I returned to my seat and did my best. When I went home that evening, my temperature was

102 degrees. When I got my paper back a few days later, I received a "B" with the comment: "This isn't bad, Betty, considering the shape you were in!"

Now as I looked around me at the busyness of this huge campus and thought of going to a linguistics class before I could go home, I faced the truth. Something was wrong. I was too tired to go on. Yet nothing I did was taking the fatigue away. I had checked with student health at the UCLA Medical Center. The result? A vitamin shot which was of negligible value! It was just the first of many vitamin shots which frustrated physicians were to use as treatment for a disease they did not know existed.

As I continued to sit and think I finally made up my mind. Denial wasn't working. I had to do something concrete to help myself. I decided that I needed to get away for the weekend. It was Friday, and IVCF, one of the Christian student groups on campus, was having a weekend retreat in the mountains. Some of my friends were going and had been trying to talk me into going too. My excuse had been that I was too tired. But now I began to believe that I should go BECAUSE I was tired. I'd probably feel great by Monday!

That evening as I sat in front of a roaring fire, listening to the inspiring words of the speaker, I began to relax. Instead of a taut feeling of exhaustion I began to feel drowsy, as though I could lie down and sleep forever. After the meeting I decided to forgo just "hanging out" and to return to our dorm-like accommodations instead and go to bed.

As everyone in that dorm straggled in later on they would wake me up, but that didn't seem to matter. I was sure I would either sleep through all the noise or rapidly fall back to sleep again.

For a few brief moments I relaxed under the blanket. This was exactly what I had needed. I felt whole again: body, mind and spirit coming together in peaceful harmony. Then just as suddenly I felt wired. I was awake, wide awake, too tired to sleep, if that makes sense! First I was tense physically, then my emotions became gripped in an escalating panic. And so the cycle went through all the hours of the night. Others went to bed, thinking I was already asleep. I made sure they kept on thinking that. After all, how could I explain how I felt?

I made many trips to the bathroom just to think. Even now, years later, I can remember the "deals" I tried to make with God if He would only get me through the night. I truly thought that I was "cracking up."

Even after no sleep, morning looked good. The world around me looked normal and the panic had left. Only the nagging fatigue reminded me of the nightmare of the last twelve hours. Now a new problem arose. I simply had to go home. Now! But no one whom I had come with was going home until Sunday. Then I had a chance encounter with a former boyfriend who wanted to leave early, early as in a few hours! To make our untimely departure even more legitimate, one of the main speakers needed a ride down the mountain in order to keep a speaking engagement on

Sunday. It all looked so normal, even sacrificial. No one knew what I was going through, and for the moment that was best.

Once home, all my parents knew was that I was tired. They were getting used to that, so they were not unduly alarmed. Meanwhile, I was slipping back into denial mode. When I was a little girl all life's problems had seemed better in the morning after a good night's sleep. This present problem would pass too. Some morning I would wake up refreshed after a night's sleep and this nightmare would have passed. "I'll be better in the morning," I reassured myself.

In reality each morning followed the previous one bringing with it more tiredness and greater fear over what was happening. I dropped all but two classes, and managed to start teaching in the fall, but the effort was agonizing. My grip on God was my greatest source of strength. My family was incredibly supportive. At the same time some who shared my faith were my greatest source of pain when they would equate my situation with lack of trust in God. When there are no known answers for human pain, some feel the need to invent their own answers, and by so doing they can cause much harm.

For twenty years I sought for a diagnosis and a cure, spiritual and psychological as well as physical. They were years of huge medical bills, a lot of medical tests and doctor searching, medical experiments, and alterations in lifestyle and careers. At times the experimentation extended to bizarre treatments, like multiple capsules of incubated animal glandular material and an injection of urine from a pregnant woman, all administered by licensed medical doctors who were simply conducting their own experiments. Needless to say, they didn't work.

At some point I dropped the search for answers and continued to adapt my lifestyle to what I could do. I had a deep belief in the fact that God does not make mistakes, and that every moment of our life has value regardless of how we feel. For that reason I could look to Him to show me how I could use all of this to do His will and help others. To paraphrase psychiatrist Viktor Frankl, he who knows the why to his existence can endure any how.

It wasn't easy, however. For 12 years I taught school and was a high school counselor. I enjoyed working with high school students almost as much as I love writing and having a private counseling practice now. That affinity for my work has helped, but some days are still excruciatingly hard to get through because of my physical exhaustion. During my teaching days a doctor ordered me to take a year of sick leave to see if that would provide a cure. Of course, it didn't, but it did start me on my writing career since I was bored and had plenty of time to write. When I went back to work that fall, however, I was as exhausted as ever. Sometimes I would lie down on my bed before work and cry, feeling that physically I just couldn't keep doing this. But there was no way out but forward.

Changing careers from teaching to psychotherapy and writing has made working possible. But every day I fight against a pervasive tiredness. Pacing has helped, as does learning to say "No," a word I never knew how to use before. Above all, God has sustained me, and family and friends are supportive. All these are adaptive tools, tools which every person with a chronic disease needs to have in their toolbox.

It was only a few years ago that a physician bluntly warned me against any renewed testing and diagnosed me as having Chronic Fatigue Syndrome, CFS, perhaps more accurately labeled CFIDS, Chronic Fatigue Immune Dysfunction Syndrome. That morning, after I had been given the diagnosis, my daughter and I went for breakfast. She was the first person with whom I shared the news. I can remember the relief I felt, the affirmation. The unknown had always seemed so nebulous, so unsure. All this pain had been real after all, as if I hadn't already believed it.

Another physician confirmed the diagnosis, and then another. I don't have any more energy because of that diagnosis, but at least now it has a name and that has made a world of difference. And every time I say "No" to exhausting labors, I don't feel that old guilt. I don't feel lazy. Maybe somewhere deep inside, until I had that label I would have always entertained a level of self doubt and self blame.

A man who runs a coffee shop nearby has a sign on his counter which reads "Never, never, never give up." It inspires me some days as I sit across from it and slowly sip my coffee. Strangely enough, I am a happy person most of the time, just tired and so tired of being tired. CFIDS has not destroyed my life, even after 50 years. It has limited the scope of some of my dreams and made each day a challenge. But sometimes it can even motivate positive action. After both musician Brenton Brown and his wife came down with CFIDS, he composed the beloved song "Everlasting God," which speaks of God's presence and enablement. Yet CFIDS is a disease which I still hope will be eradicated from the face of the earth someday soon.

NOTES

NOTES

What Is Chronic Fatigue Syndrome?

When I began to have the symptoms of CFIDS, way back during my UCLA days, I can remember an almost panicky feeling of "Push harder, push harder. Prove it isn't real!" Of course, pushing harder only made it worse and also increased my anxiety level. The futility of this approach reached its peak during a game of tennis. I was as able to play tennis as I was able to run a marathon; I just didn't know that yet.

It was a lovely summer evening when a friend and I went to a local school where we could use their tennis court. Years before, my Uncle Dave had taught me how to play tennis and I had loved it ever since. I hadn't played for a while, however, not since I had developed the symptoms of CFIDS.

For a few minutes I played vigorously. It felt good to be physically active again. But then it was all over. My leg muscles became weak, and I felt shaky and exhausted. I could barely stand on legs which felt like jelly and were actually giving out. John half carried me to the car where I eventually regained enough muscular strength to walk into my house once we arrived there. I never played tennis again. It was only the first of many activities which had to be reluctantly abandoned.

Just what is Chronic Fatigue Syndrome? Even the label Chronic Fatigue Syndrome has been under debate and is only one of many names given to this disease. In today's literature you will often find it listed as ME/CFS, ME/CFIDS, or just CFIDS, "chronic fatigue/immune dysfunction syndrome," as opposed to CFS alone. In that way it combines "the symptom of fatigue with the presence of immune system markers, thus separating it from generic chronic fatigue."[1] ME stands for myalgic encephalomyelitis and is the term used in the U.K. According to the *Journal of Internal Medicine*:

> The label "chronic fatigue syndrome" (CFS) has persisted for many years because of lack of knowledge of the etiological agents and of the disease process. In view of more recent research and clinical experience that strongly point to widespread inflammation and multisystemic neuropathology, it is more appropriate and correct to use the term "myalgic encephalomyelitis" (ME) because it includes an underlying pathophysiology. It is also consistent with the neurological classification of ME in the World Health Organization's International Classification of Diseases (ICD G93.3).[2]

Whatever you call it, most basically CFIDS is characterized by a devastating fatigue to which the tiredness normally felt after a long day of work doesn't even begin to relate in severity. Furthermore, while lack of sleep will make it worse, sleep in itself does not take away the exhaustion. A person with CFIDS usually wakes up tired. In addition, if the person with CFIDS exerts himself physically, or even emotionally, the negative results can be felt as long as 24 hours or more later and the resultant fatigue will not go away "after a good night's sleep." Usually at least a day or more are required for "recovery" back to the more usual exhausted state.

Other symptoms can include:

- Cognitive problems, "brain fog"
- Sore throat
- Enlarged lymph nodes in neck or armpits
- Unexplained muscle pain
- Low-grade fever
- Abdominal problems
- Anxiety or depression
- Tinnitus (ringing in ears)

According to the CDC,

> The primary symptom of CFS is unexplained, severe fatigue lasting at least 6 months that is not improved by bed rest and that can get worse after physical activity or mental exertion. Individuals with CFS experience a fatigue so strong that their activity levels and stamina decline dramatically. However, fatigue is not

the only symptom, and for some patients may not be the symptom that bothers them the most.

As stated in the 1994 case definition, the fatigue of CFS is accompanied by at least 4 of 8 characteristic symptoms lasting at least 6 months. These symptoms include:

- post-exertion malaise lasting more than 24 hours
- unrefreshing sleep
- significant impairment of short-term memory or concentration
- muscle pain
- pain in the joints without swelling or redness
- headaches of a new type, pattern, or severity
- tender lymph nodes in the neck or armpit
- a sore throat that is frequent or recurring

The symptoms listed above are the symptoms used to diagnose this illness. However, many CFS patients may experience other symptoms, including irritable bowel, depression or other psychological problems, chills and night

sweats, visual disturbances, brain fog, difficulty
maintaining upright position, dizziness, balance
problems, fainting, and allergies or sensitivities
to foods, odors, chemicals, medications, or
noise.[3]

To summarize Dr. Jose Montoya of Stanford, it is
sometimes said that "CFS is another form of death." To
him that description explains why people who are helped
by him often exclaim, "Thank you for giving me back my
life."[4]

Yet CFIDS varies in severity from person to person.
Laura Hillenbrand, the best-selling author of *Seabiscuit: An
American Legend* and, more recently, *Unbroken: A World
War II Story of Survival, Resilience, and Redemption*, went
from being a very athletic person to a state where she
could not even sit up, all in a few days. After that she was
bedridden for two years. Laura became ill with CFIDS at
19. Diagnosed at Johns Hopkins, she compares the term
"chronic fatigue" to what she feels as "fatigue," to be like
comparing "a match ... to an atomic bomb."[5]

At the other end of the spectrum there are many people
who function on a somewhat normal schedule with a
low-grade pervasive discomfort. Then there are various
gradations of function and discomfort/pain in between.
From person to person it varies. And even within one person
the symptoms are not completely predictable. Some days
are better or worse. Even certain years seem better or worse
than others. With the new definition of ME, however,

symptom severity must result in a 50 percent or greater reduction of a patient's premorbid activity level.[6] (See chart at end of booklet under Resources.)

The hypotheses as to cause as well as treatment of CFIDS vary almost as much as the symptoms. In a good summary of the history of the causes of CFIDS, Dr. David S. Bell, MD, FAAP, reports that in the 1950's it was believed to be an infectious disease. After that it was relegated to psychiatry – probably depression or hysteria. That label lasted for a few years and still lingers on in the minds of some. But then psychiatry has far too often been a dumping ground for whatever conventional medicine cannot diagnose and/ or cure! In my opinion, CFIDS may well be responsible for many of those Victorian women who were said to have the vapors! After psychiatry, according to Dr. Bell, CFIDS was felt to be an endocrine disease; then because of bowel symptoms, an illness of the gastrointestinal tract. Since the 1990's the focus has turned unsuccessfully to the brain.

According to Dr. Bell, it has become increasingly obvious that CFIDS "is not an organ-specific illness; it is not localized in a single organ system." Rather than organs, adds Bell, "we need to change the focus of our telescope from looking at large organs to looking at single cells."[7]

According to the CDC,

> Despite a vigorous search, scientists have not yet identified what causes CFS. While a single cause for CFS may yet be identified, another possibility is that CFS has multiple triggers.

Some of the possible causes of CFS might be:

- infections
- immune dysfunction
- abnormally low blood pressure that can cause fainting (neurally mediated hypotension)
- nutritional deficiency
- stress that activates the axis where the hypothalamus, pituitary, and adrenal glands interact (the HPA axis)[8]

It is the year 2015 at the time of my writing this booklet. I have now had CFIDS for more than 50 years. Once I realized that there was no cure forthcoming, I kept distantly in touch with any new possibilities for treatment, but I've never gone back to the intense doctor searching and testing of those earlier days. Having the disease labeled, and knowing that it is a disease, helped me to go on in spite of no real treatment. Fortunately I can, with difficulty, function enough to work.

In recent years came XMRV, a specific retrovirus. That brought new hope. For me it created a period of "catch up," just to make sure I wasn't missing some new explanation or treatment for CFIDS. I wasn't, not really, and interest in XMRV died down. There are studies which indicate that CFIDS may be a result of the body's immune system reacting to an invading virus. If so, such a reaction could cause CFIDS-like symptoms.

However, a generally pervasive view of the cause of CFIDS

is that it often follows a bout of some virus or bacterial infection, something like the flu. It has been noted that with an outbreak of the flu, for example, long after most of those affected have recovered, certain individuals may linger on with symptoms which can then morph into CFIDS. It seems possible that the difference lies in genetics. In that case who would go on to get CFIDS would be determined by the host response, meaning genetic factors which support the illness.

The genetic factor is of particular interest to me. Back in those college years another incident is etched into my mind. I can still remember, with vivid detail, standing at the top of the stairs leading into Kerkhoff Hall waiting for my boyfriend. We were serious about marriage, but for me a dark cloud was forming. I was not well. That I was sure of, even if no doctor could figure it out! I wanted children – four would be ideal or maybe at least two: Katherine Elizabeth and Edward Emanuel to be exact! But what if I had a genetic disorder? What if I gave this horrible exhaustion to these children? Did I have the right to drag a husband into that dilemma?

Although I carried those fears too far, since it is not that predictable that my children would have been affected, according to those who believe in the genetic factor usually someone who has CFIDS can point to at least one other person in their family tree who also has CFIDS. So my fears had some reasonable foundation.

Later on, long before I was actually diagnosed with

CFIDS, the genetic question mark came up once again in my thinking. My Aunt Esther had always been a favorite of mine. She was old enough to be my mother's mother but was delightfully active and fun. She loved to cook and was the perfect hostess. If someone would tell her to stop and rest for a while, she would quip: "Sit down? I can't sit down! I just got to Heaven and I've got to look around." Then with that twinkle in her eye, she'd carry on with her task. She loved life and people.

Suddenly in later life, overnight she slumped into total exhaustion. She began to sound like me and we both recognized it. Neither of us knew why, and both of us got our vitamin shots which didn't help. She never recovered. When she was on her deathbed, most of our family was gathered in her room. She looked up at me with love and a bit of her old twinkle and said her last words to me: "Elizabeth understands!" There is a community in shared suffering.

In 2010 the American Red Cross requested people diagnosed with CFIDS to abstain from donating blood. Other countries have made the same request. Both Stanford and Columbia now include CFIDs in their Infectious Disease Departments. In some perverse way such actions have helped to validate the existence of CFIDS as a disease.

At least one other area of focus which is currently being studied as to its relationship to CFIDS is the "cortisol awakening response." Cortisol is a secretion of the adrenal gland and has a profound affect on bodily functions. Women and men, with and without a CFIDS diagnosis, were tested for cortisol levels upon awakening and 30 and 60 minutes after awakening. Women with CFIDS had significantly lower levels of cortisol upon awakening, unlike other women not diagnosed with CFIDS and unlike all men tested. This test result may help explain why women more than men get CFIDS.[9]

As a lay person with CFIDS it causes me to wonder if my usual awakening feeling of painful exhaustion may be related to low cortisol levels and why, when I get out of bed after forcing myself to lie there awake for a short time, that eases the jump from sleep to awakening. Since it is believed that cortisol is elevated by coffee, I may also have an explanation as to why, when I am out of bed and drink that first cup of coffee, I begin to feel a little more energetic. At that point I can usually continue on with the day as opposed to the feeling of I just can't do it at all. It's just an hypothesis, but then again so much about CFIDS is more hypothesis than absolute fact.

The good news is that at least most people now see CFIDS as a viable disorder. Definition and especially cause and cure are still lacking in answers. But the visibility it has gained in recent years has boosted funds donated and a desire to perform a level of research which will someday give us more definitive answers. To many of us "someday" sounds way off. Unless we are very young, it many not happen, at least completely, in our time.

Certain palliative approaches are at times used to give a small margin of relief to the symptoms of CFIDS: everything from B_{12} or calcium injections to the selective, carefully chosen use of certain antidepression medications. With CFIDS some people suffer from a somewhat relaxed but profound exhaustion while others experience a more agitated fatigue. For the latter, even an antidepressant, like Prozac or Wellbutrin, which acts as a stimulant will usually not help since it will ease the fatigue but at the same time possibly exacerbate the tension. Similarly, drugs like Provigil, Nuvigil or Symmetrel have seemed to offer a source of added energy for some. At the same time, the cure as well as the cause have so far been lacking.

Dr. David Bell is an expert in Chronic Fatigue Syndrome as a result of observing first hand a group of patients involved in an outbreak in 1985 in Lyndonville, New York. Because he was so closely involved with these people as their personal physician, he speaks with confidence about the struggles of those of us who go on in spite of CFIDS. For a long time people who had CFIDS were ignored by the medical community, partly because most providers didn't know what to do and were threatened by their own lack of effectiveness. "Without a medical provider to look after the ... patient, the world becomes more harsh and cruel, as if the illness were not bad enough to start with."[10] Ignorance and denial of the validity of CFIDS still exists even in the medical community but not as much as before; and out and out denial is more tentative now. Many providers just don't know much about CFIDS.

The worst case scenario is to be told by that medical provider that your tests are negative and so there is nothing wrong with you. Usually the expectation seems to be that normal tests should make you feel happy. Therefore, sometimes you fake it and act happy so you won't look like some weird person who wants to be sick. But inside you'd rather have a truly bad diagnosis if it would validate to others and yourself how badly you feel. You try so hard to keep going, but can never quite push hard enough to look like everyone else. Above all, without a positive test result, how can you hope for effective treatment?

After they give you the "good" news about your test results, the practitioner may add that you look healthy, so there's nothing more that they or anyone else can do – except, of course, to send you to a shrink! But, says Dr. Bell: "Being told to go away and see someone else, maybe a psychiatrist, is devastating for the patient. ... They would rather be told that they have a possibly fatal neurological disease, believe it or not. It is an illustration of the importance of illness validation by a medical provider."[11] That is why to have at least CFIDS as a name of a disorder, a real diagnosis which can be looked up and found in a Google search or on the NIH website, at least helps the emotional health of those of us who have it.

NOTES

NOTES

Coping With CFIDS

Right before I was diagnosed with CFIDS, a physician told me that I did not have the physical strength to work. That was when I was still in my early twenties. My reaction was typical for me. To tell me I was unable to do something was to catapult me into doing it. I would pace, I decided. I would give up some activities. I would stay in bed one day a week if needed. But quit? Never!

How to do this became the challenge, however. Even after the diagnosis of Chronic Fatigue Syndrome is given, since both cause and cure are still at this point in time unknown, building spiritual, emotional and physical strength in all ways possible is essential. With CFIDS, for example, you can't afford to lose sleep or skip meals. Furthermore, emotionally and spiritually, without a relationship with Jesus Christ my journey would be very difficult. God's promise, "I will never leave you nor forsake you" (Hebrews 13:5), is more than just a nice platitude. The Old Testament affirmation, "Shall not the Judge of all the earth do right?" (Genesis 18:25) is my answer to "Why me?"

God doesn't always say "Yes" to our requests – or "No," for that matter. He says either and sometimes He says "Wait." The "name it and claim it" game is not biblical.

God's answers to our prayers are His answers, not ours.

If anyone deserved a "Yes" answer to a cure for his "thorn in the flesh," Paul did. Yet after three pleas for healing a condition which most biblical scholars feel related to Paul's fading eyesight, the answer remained "No." But there was always God's supply. Paul's response can provide great encouragement to all of us: "Since I know it is all for Christ's good, I am quite happy about 'the thorn,' and about insults and hardships, persecutions and difficulties; for when I am weak, then I am strong – the less I have, the more I depend on him." (II Corinthians 12:10)

In addition to the biblical resources which exist, for me pacing became an essential tool. What does it mean to pace? Perhaps the best way for me to explain how I have handled that issue is to take as an example a major time of the year when both demands and expectations are heightened. For me that time is Christmas. I figure if I can pace my life at Christmas, I can apply those principles of behavior to life in general.

When I was growing up, Christmas was always the most magical time of the year. As a Swedish immigrant family, we followed the tradition of having our main celebration on Christmas Eve. In preparation my mother baked coffee cake and seven or eight different kinds of Christmas cookies. She made Swedish potato sausage from scratch, while my father spent several days chopping onions, squeezing lemons, and deboning herring in preparation for his yearly contribution to the Christmas festivities, his own special pickled herring.

This he prepared for our family celebration as well as for gifts for bank tellers, grocery clerks and a variety of people he encountered throughout the year. It was a tradition everyone loved.

On our door hung a wreath of pine boughs and holly made by my mother. More greenery and candles adorned the mantle, while the meaning of Christmas, the birth of the Christ child, was portrayed in a nativity scene on the buffet in the dining room. In the living room, under the lighted tree, miniature figures formed a small village on the white cotton snow.

On Christmas Eve the relatives all came with their bags of wrapped presents which were added to those gifts already under the tree. With typical childhood avarice we children waited for all the food to be eaten and the inevitable dishwashing to be accomplished so that we could finally open these mysterious packages. Duplicating such a childhood Christmas would be a hard act for anyone to follow. Today, with the demands of blended families trying to have two or three separate celebrations in one day, it is even harder, to the point where Christmas and, indeed, any holiday can become a negative experience instead of the joyous time it is meant to be.

Choosing some different ways of doing things is the key for survival. In that context, choice means taking control over the stress and chaos of unrealistic demands and expectations, according to your own level of energy at any given time, even those demands which are self imposed by your own desires or sense of guilt. The following are some suggestions on how to cope more effectively and even enjoy Christmas or any other holiday or special event.

1. Declare your boundaries, politely but firmly. Try not to go to multiple events in one day or maybe even in one weekend. Don't over explain. People in general will not understand the word "tired" beyond their own experiences. Most of the time it is probably wise to simply say, "I am unable to come, but I appreciate your invitation," rather than, "I'm too tired."

2. Don't compare yourself with others. Accept your limitations without blaming or hating yourself. Also realize that those people you know who seem to be able to do it all aren't always doing as well as they appear. In my counseling office I see people whose personal lives may be falling apart while they rush around to all the activities of the season.

3. For many of us, buying and wrapping presents are the final stressers that feel like just too much. Shopping early, using home shopping on TV or the Internet, wrapping ahead of time, using bags rather than wrapping paper, and getting help from a teenager or friend are all ways to relieve some of the stress. Last year I found a wrapping set with boxes, pre-cut paper with tear-off strips which enabled the paper to stick, tags,

and other decorative items. Look for these kinds of shortcuts. For example, QVC online or on television is a good source which can be accessed right in your home.

4. If the stress is greater than usual, due to an illness or extra family or business demands, cut down on your decorating expectations. Choose a favorite decoration rather than decorating your entire house inside and out. Focus on a tree and wreath or create a Christmas village scene. Save some things for another year. If you alternate decorations rather than using them all at one time, the stress will be less and the change will add variety to other Christmases.

5. Think of simple ways to entertain, like dessert instead of a full dinner or take in food from a deli arranged attractively on festive dishes. Be more casual and serve buffet. Let people help you serve and clean up. And above all, plan ahead by freezing foods instead of cooking at the last minute.

6. Develop your own secrets to simplify entertaining. If you serve a full meal, focus on one special entrée and simplify the rest. Aim for simple elegance. For example, if you want to make a complicated dish, like homemade bread or a special casserole, do it ahead of time and freeze it. Then serve it with a frozen vegetable or green salad.

7. Create a favorite dish which is easy to make but

impressive in looks and taste. Use it often as something you can count on. One time when I was trying to blend simplicity with elegance, I made a dessert I called Berry Swirl. I simply put alternate layers of vanilla ice cream, whipped cream, and raspberries in parfait glasses, topping them with a dollop of whipped cream and a berry and adding a teaspoon of berry juice on the top so it could drip down. Then I put the glasses in the freezer until twenty minutes before serving. The first time I used this dessert one of the best, most energetic cooks I know fell in love with it and asked for the recipe, calling it my "mousse." It was an awkward moment!

8. Try creative ways to entertain which do the work for you. Let each guest bring a dish, but organize their choices so there will be variety. Or have a Christmas tree decorating party and serve dessert. A similar plan can work with a Christmas card writing party. Use card tables and have each person bring their cards, writing materials, and a finger food snack for everyone else. Keep it small though.

9. In between the activities, maintain better nutrition as stress increases. Protein snacks, fresh vegetables and fruits, combined with less sugar and fats, can help in maintaining your energy level during the holidays. And don't forget to keep hydrated.

10. Plan your rest time as much as your activities. Space your events so that active days are followed by those which have less demands. Do something inspirational. Spend some time with a good friend. Listen to Handel's *Messiah* while you enjoy the lights on your tree and sip some eggnog.

For those who experienced Christmas as a time of pure joy in childhood, adult holidays may seem unable to compete. In contrast, past memories may evoke feelings of loneliness for what was.

Yet for those who never had happy holidays in their past, occasions like Christmas, Hanukkah and even birthdays may bring feelings of sadness over what never was or what might have been. In essence, either way holidays like Christmas can then be a trigger for depression.

Whether we are haunted by what used to be or by what never was, once we learn to make some practical changes to reduce holiday stress, then the way to having a happier holiday is to cut the old tapes of the past and focus forward. As Ruth Bell Graham said so frequently in our conversations, "Make the least of all that goes and the most of all that comes." The same principle holds true for the celebration of any special occasion and even for more everyday occasions.

The year that Christmas was only a reminder of a fatal car accident which had recently taken my mother's life and changed my own life forever, my survival at Christmas was greatly helped by trying to provide a Christmas celebration for some foster children, rather than seeking much pleasure for myself. I had to leave the past and go on. And it worked. I gave myself a break from all the "Ho! Ho! Ho!" aspects of traditional holiday celebration. I made sure I got enough rest. Then for several hours on Christmas day I forgot about *me* and focused on *them*. Before I knew it, Christmas was over and something good had happened after all. I gave a little to a few deprived and abused kids and got so much more back in terms of healing.

Sometimes we do more by doing less. Don't be afraid to say "No" to exhausting demands, and choose to celebrate occasions in whatever unique way is right for you. You and everyone around you may actually have greater enjoyment as a result of not trying so hard to make it "perfect." At Christmas, put God back as the focus of your Christmas and remember once again what the season is really all about.

With CFIDS, and with most chronic diseases which limit activity, pacing is an essential tool. Plan ahead, but plan realistically. During that last semester at UCLA, I wrote out a schedule, but it was far from realistic. I could fit in a full schedule of classes and other activities, like a teaching assistant job, leadership in a campus organization, and church. They were all written into small, orderly boxes. But there was no room for a car repair or a bout of the flu, or making meals or dating, which all happened whether I organized them into my schedule or not. On dating, for example, "We'll just go out for a Coke and come back," I'd rationalize. But then the fatigue would hit and plans would change.

First of all, the schedule only worked on paper, not in real life, *even* if there were no unplanned interruptions! In real life the expectations were even too heavy for a healthy normal person *without* CFIDS. So I was doomed to failure to start with! Add emergencies and unexpected demands to that and no one could have followed the schedule. Once again plan, pace, but do it realistically.

When you plan a schedule, be honest with yourself and others. If you want friends, don't belabor your symptoms. But, on the other hand, when you can't go out for dinner on a given night because you want to make it to work the next day, admit that to yourself and politely decline. If feelings get hurt, then you may have to explain why. Your real friends will understand.

In some ways accommodating CFIDS is not that different from dealing with any other chronic disease – except for the stigma that sometimes accompanies its vague definition, cause and cure. If you have degenerative disc disease, for example, and drop a pen on the floor, you may need to ask someone to bend over and pick it up and they will understand your back pain. If you have osteoarthritis you definitely will not be a mountain climber. That fact will be obvious. Simply said, anyone with a chronic disease may at times need help and may have to opt out of certain activities. CFIDS is no different from some of these other conditions which limit activity except that it is not always understood. Because sometimes people believe that CFIDS is just plain old-fashioned tiredness, it may be necessary to explain the difference. Above all, don't let the skepticism of some who still remain ignorant of the disease cause you to doubt yourself and feel lazy or guilty.

A favorite writer of mine, Amy Carmichael, once wrote the words: "In acceptance lieth peace." Fight for a cure. Get treatment when it's there. But for now, and even then, acceptance and going forth with your life is the best way to handle a chronic disease. Pace, but never give up.

NOTES

NOTES

The Miracle of Choice

A psychiatrist-friend of mine was dying of cancer, but as long as his body could be forced to do so, he and a friend would go down by the ocean and, with great difficulty for him, explore a ship or two and in general "hang out." Often they ended up at a coffee shop. My friend could barely eat, but the ambiance created by coffee and good friendship was relaxing.

One day a man joined them at a sort of communal table. He looked disheveled and tired. "Life sucks," he muttered to himself as he stirred his coffee. "Don't you think it sucks?" he asked as he turned to my friend. Quickly he went on. "I've lost my job, my kid's failing in school, and my wife is a nag. I'd say life sucks!"

Pulling himself painfully out of the fatigue which had brought my friend and his companion to stop at this coffee shop in the first place, my friend gave all of his attention to the desperate man they had just met.

"No, life doesn't suck at all," he responded. "It can be rough, even painful. It can seem hopeless. But every minute of life is a miracle. Every moment has meaning. Man, you've got to find out what's really important about life. You may not have a job, but you have a life. Your kid may be a lazy bum right now, but you have a kid. Maybe your wife feels like you do. Find out! Ask her! Embrace what you have. Stop running!"

At that point my friend needed to leave the ocean retreat and go home before he collapsed, but he left behind a man who smiled and thanked him as he left, a man who never knew he had just had a free session with a pricey psychiatrist, much less a man who would be dead in a couple of weeks.

Besides alterations in lifestyle and good nutrition, fundamental to transcending the crippling results of CFIDS is our attitude toward it. "Every life, in every situation and to the last breath, has a meaning, retains a meaning. This is equally true of the life of a sick person, even the mentally sick. *The so-called life not worth living does not exist.*"[12]

Once again we can endure any how if we know the why. Psychiatrist Viktor Frankl wrote after his losses and torture in Hitler's death camps: "... *man should not ask what he may expect from life, but should rather understand that life expects something from him.* ... Life is a task," a task which requires choice and action.[13]

> The night before her leg was to be amputated for tuberculosis of the bone, another patient wrote a letter to a friend hinting at thoughts of suicide. The letter was intercepted and fell into the hands of a doctor in the surgical ward where this patient lay. The doctor lost no time, but found a pretext for a talk with the woman. In a few appropriate words he too pointed out

to the patient that human life would be a very poor thing indeed if the loss of a leg actually involved depriving it of all meaning. Such a loss could at most make the life of an ant purposeless since it would no longer be able to achieve the goal set for it by the ant community – namely, running around on all six legs and being useful. For a human being it must be different. The young doctor's chat with the woman, couched rather in the style of a Socratic dialogue, did not fail to take effect. His senior surgeon, who undertook the amputation next morning, does not know to this day that in spite of the successful operation this patient almost ended up on his autopsy table.[14]

Both the physician and the patient made choices and then acted according to those choices. The stakes were high: life or death.

Frankl's attitude toward life was that under any condition, under any adverse circumstance, even chronic disease, life has meaning. From a biblical point of view the psalmist tells us: "You saw me before I was born and scheduled each day of my life before I began to breathe. Every day was recorded in your Book." (Psalm 140:16, *The Living Bible*) God calls the shots on when our lives end. The end time is not ours to choose for ourselves or anyone else; and as long as God decides to keep us here our lives have meaning.

Sometimes having meaning involves the joy of knowing

God in a very deep and real way. Last week I had a day where I felt too weak to go on. One hour into my day, with four hours to go, I felt an increasingly overwhelming fatigue.

In circumstances where I have felt my own inadequacy to love someone who is unlovable, or to be patient with an irritating circumstance, I have sometimes sent up a fast SOS to God: "Your love, Lord," or "Your patience." The feelings don't usually change at that very moment, but as I go forward and act in love, the feelings of love begin to be felt. These actions involve choice. The rest is up to God.

On that day last week I tried this technique on a physical level: "Your strength, Lord." As I went through my day, I forgot about that prayer until three hours before my work for that day was finished. Suddenly it occurred to me that I felt better than usual. I had close to normal strength, whatever that is! By the end of the day, I became more tired again, but I was still able to shop for a few groceries at a nearby market.

Then I remembered the quick prayer I had uttered, and also a hymn which I hadn't heard for years. It was written as a poem by Annie Johnson Flint, a woman who knew the pain and frustration of chronic illness. When she developed rheumatoid arthritis in her teen years she was soon unable to walk. She had wanted to be a concert pianist, but the RA soon put an end to that aspiration. She could, however, still compose, even if it meant typing with her knuckles because of her swollen joints! One of these compositions was, "He

Giveth More Grace as the Burdens Grow Greater." One line in that poem stood out to me as I remembered and reread the poem: "When our strength has failed ere the day is half done ... "

My strength had failed "ere the day was half done." But then there was God. Some days are just plain hard and relief seems far away. But a small miracle last week not only helped me through an extra tiring day; it refreshed my faith in God and His concern in even the small details of life. And on that day my tiredness and its relief felt much bigger than a small detail!

In Frankl's terminology, we may not always be able to choose our circumstances, *however* we can choose our attitude toward them. We can choose to go on. In another example, when I needed physical therapy four times a week after a rotator cuff tear, the time spent in just lying there with either heat or ice packs amounted to over an hour each day. Boredom, which has always been hard for me to handle, was added to the physical pain. From the ER next door to me I could hear kids crying, and in general these hours of heating and icing were the worst times during the therapy.

Then it occurred to me that I could use the time as a specifically structured period to pray. Two people came to mind who were in particular need, and so I made a commitment within myself to use the time praying for them. I chose my meaning for that specific time of the day, rather than drift through the hour only to view it as wasted time.

A theologian from the past, F. B. Meyer, once wrote: "The will is the final expression of our personality. We are not what we feel or think or wish for: we are what we choose, determine, will."[15] It is choice which can make a major difference in dealing with CFIDS or any other chronic disease.

CFIDS presents a fatigue which is tantamount to pain. At the outset of a fatigue-provoking situation, one can determine to make it through. But at some point, if the expectations are too high, one is forced to stop from the sheer pain of forcing against that level of fatigue. To live with CFIDS is tough. Yet at this point in time, for some of us it is an unalterable circumstance of our lives. There are worse diseases than CFIDS. And within the CFIDS spectrum, some of us function at a higher level than others. But the fatigue of CFIDS is indisputably painful for all who have it. Without meaning, life can seem wasted when it is lived with this debilitating disease. Yet in contrast to that way of thinking, to waste life, when it costs so much, is indeed a tragedy. That is why a major condition of handling CFIDS is to choose to find meaning in it.

Life has meaning at every level of existence, and meaning has a powerful impact on those who possess it. Those who lost their sense of meaning in Hitler's camps died. In contrast,

> Goethe worked seven years on the completion of the second part of *Faust*. Finally, in January 1832, he sealed the manuscript; two months

later he died. I dare say that during the final
seven years of his life he biologically lived
beyond his means. His death was overdue, but
he remained alive up to the moment his work
was completed and meaning fulfilled.[16]

Above all, there is the ultimate quote of Viktor Frankl:
"God is not dead ... not even 'after Auschwitz'. ... "[17]

Suffering can make us into monsters or saints. Because of
suffering we can understand another's pain; we can develop
a deeper relationship with God. Who do people turn to
when they hurt? Think about it. Do you really want the
comfort and advice of someone who has never suffered?
No, most of us rely on people who "get it," who understand
pain.

A child lying on the operating table suddenly stopped the
anesthesiologist as he began to prepare her for a surgery she
had endured many times before. "Wait!" she cried. "I need
to tell you something."

Relieved that her cry had not been one of pain, the young
doctor stopped what he was doing and waited.

"I may not live through the surgery this time," the child
said with an attitude of wisdom beyond her eight years.
"I don't want you to blame yourself. I'll be okay. I'll be in
Heaven with Jesus." Then after a long pause, full of emotion
for the physician, she added, "You can go ahead now."

A few hours later the child was in Heaven with Jesus.
Back on earth the devastated doctor wanted to find the
source of strength which had so remarkably sustained the

child, and he ultimately found it in a relationship with Jesus Christ.

The value of a life is not measured in time but in eternity. The Bible says: " ... one day is with the Lord as a thousand years, and a thousand years as one day." (II Peter 3:8) It is therefore impossible to gauge the value of a human life by the estimated number of remaining years or its presumed quality of life. Only God knows the value of His creation.

This child found the ultimate meaning in suffering, to know God. She made the choice to connect with Him and to use that connection to reach out to her physician. At her young age she had suffered with a painful chronic disease for a lifetime and had used it to draw closer to God and to her fellow man. It's not the length nor the depth of our suffering which counts, it's what we choose to do with it that matters. In the words of Russian novelist Dostoevski: "There is only one thing that I dread: not to be worthy of my sufferings."[18]

NOTES

NOTES

Epilogue

Speaking of the idea of the sovereignty of God in the existence of each of our lives, Spurgeon says: "Our presence on earth in this day of grace was a matter altogether beyond our control. ... The *continuance* of life is equally determined by God. He who fixed our birth has measured the interval between the cradle and the grave, and it shall not be a day longer or a day shorter than the divine degree. How many times your lungs shall heave and your pulses beat have been fixed by the eternal calculator from of old. What reflections ought to arise out of this! How willing we should be to labour on, even if we be weary, since God appoints our day and will not over-weary us, for he is no hard taskmaster. How glad we ought to be even to suffer if the Lord so ordains. ... The Lord's time is best: to a hair's breadth thy span of life is rightly measured. God ordains all: therefore peace, restless spirit, and let the Lord have his way."[19]

– Charles Spurgeon

CFIDS Disability Scale

100: No symptoms at rest; no symptoms with exercise; normal overall activity level; able to work full-time without difficulty.

90: No symptoms at rest; mild symptoms with activity; normal overall activity level; able to work full-time without difficulty.

80: Mild symptoms at rest; symptoms worsened by exertion; minimal activity restriction noted for activities requiring exertion only; able to work full-time with difficulty in jobs requiring exertion.

70: Mild symptoms at rest; some daily activity limitation clearly noted. Overall functioning close to 90% of expected except for activities requiring exertion. Able to work full-time with difficulty.

60: Mild to moderate symptoms at rest; daily activity limitation clearly noted. Overall functioning 70%-90%. Unable to work full-time in jobs requiring physical labor, but able to work full-time in light activity if hours flexible.

50: Moderate symptoms at rest. Moderate to severe symptoms with exercise or activity; overall activity level reduced to 70% of expected. Unable to perform strenuous duties, but able to perform light duty or desk work 4-5 hours a day, but requires rest periods.

40: Moderate symptoms at rest. Moderate to severe symptoms with exercise or activity; overall activity level reduced to 50%-70% of expected. Not confined to house. Unable to perform strenuous duties; able to perform light duty or desk work 3-4 hours a day, but requires rest periods.

30: Moderate to severe symptoms at rest. Severe symptoms with any exercise; overall activity level reduced to 50% of expected. Usually confined to house. Unable to perform any strenuous tasks. Able to perform desk work 2-3 hours a day, but requires rest periods.

20: Moderate to severe symptoms at rest. Unable to perform strenuous activity; overall activity 30%-50% of expected. Unable to leave house except rarely; confined to bed most of day; unable to concentrate for more than 1 hour a day.

10: Severe symptoms at rest; bedridden the majority of the time. No travel outside of the house. Marked cognitive symptoms preventing concentration.

0: Severe symptoms on a continuous basis; bedridden constantly; unable to care for self.

* Used by permission of David S. Bell, M.D.[20]

NOTES

NOTES

Resources

Books

Bell, David S., M.D. *The Doctor's Guide to Chronic Fatigue Syndrome*. Da Capo Press, 1995.

Bell, David S., M.D., FAAP. *Cellular Hypoxia and Neuro-Immune Fatigue*. Livermore, CA: WingSpan Press, 2007.

Campbell, Bruce F., Ph.D. *The CFIDS/Fibromyalgia Toolkit: A Practical Self-Help Guide*. San Jose: Authors Choice Press, 2001.

Frankl, Viktor E., M.D., Ph.D. *Man's Search for Meaning*. Boston: Beacon Press, 2006.

Lewis, C. S. *The Problem of Pain*. New York: HarperCollins, 2001.

Skoglund, Elizabeth. *Divine Recycling: Living Above Your Circumstances*. Burbank: Netmenders, 2010.

Skoglund, Elizabeth. *Found Faithful: The Timeless Stories of Charles Spurgeon, Amy Carmichael, C.S. Lewis, Ruth Bell Graham, and Others*. Grand Rapids: Discovery House Publishers, 2003.

Ten Boom, Corrie, with Elizabeth and John Sherrill. *The*

Hiding Place. Grand Rapids,: Chosen Books, 2006.

Wilson, James L., ND, DC, Ph.D. *Adrenal Fatigue: The 21st Century Stress Syndrome*. Petaluma, CA: Smart Publications, 2001.

Websites

CFIDS Association of America – www.cfids.org

Elizabeth. R. Skoglund – www.elizabethskoglund.com

Footnotes

1. David S. Bell, M.D., *The Doctor's Guide to Chronic Fatigue Syndrome* (Da Capo Press, 1995), 1.
2. B. M. Carruthers, M. I. van de Sande, K. L. De Meirleir, N. G. Klimas, G. Broderick, T. Mitchell, D. Staines, A. C. P. Powles, N. Speight, R. Vallings, L. Bateman, B. Baumgarten-Austrheim, D. S. Bell, N. Carlo-Stella, J. Chia, A. Darragh, D. Jo, D. Lewis, A. R. Light, S. Marshall-Gradisbik, I. Mena, J. A. Mikovits, K. Miwa, M. Murovska, M. L. Pall, and S. Stevens, "Myalgic encephalomyelitis: International Consensus Criteria." *Journal of Internal Medicine.* doi: 10.1111/j.1365-2796.2011.02428.x (2011), 1.
3. http://www.cdc.gov/cfs/general/, "Chronic Fatigue Syndrome (CFS): General Information," Centers for Disease Control and Prevention. Web. May 14, 2012.
4. http://www.youtube.com/watch?v=cZntAs_isEw&feature=player_embedded, StanfordHospital, "Chronic Fatigue Syndrome: Stanford Medical Minutes with Dr. Montoya." YouTube. Web. April 11, 2011.

5. Tara Parker-Pope, "An Author Escapes From Chronic Fatigue Syndrome," *The New York Times* (February 4, 2011), http://well.blogs.nytimes.com/2011/02/04/an-author-escapes-from-chronic-fatigue-syndrome/?emc=eta1.

6. Carruthers et al. "Myalgic encephalomyelitis: International Consensus Criteria" 2.

7. David S. Bell M.D., FAAP, *Cellular Hypoxia and Neuro-Immune Fatigue* (Livermore, CA: WingSpan Press, 2007), 2.

8. Centers for Disease Control and Prevention.

9. Urs M. Nater, Elizabeth Maloney, Roumiana S. Boneva, Brian M. Gurbaxani, Jin-Mann Lin, James F. Jones, William C. Reeves, and Christine Heim, "Attenuated Morning Salivary Cortisol Concentrations in a Population-based Study of Persons with Chronic Fatigue Syndrome and Well Controls," *Journal of Clinical Endocrinol Metabolism*, March 2008, 93(3): 703.

10. Bell *Cellular Hypoxia* 1.

11. Bell *Cellular Hypoxia* 26.

12. Viktor E. Frankl, M.D., Ph.D., *Anthology*, edited, outlined, and annotated by Timothy Lent (Xlibris, 2004), 146.

13. Viktor E. Frankl, M.D., Ph.D., *The Doctor and the Soul: From Psychotherapy to Logotherapy* (New York: Vintage Books, 1973), xv.

14. Frankl *Doctor* 283.

15. F. B. Meyer, D.D., *The Call and Challenge of the Unseen* (London: Marshall, Morgan & Scott, Ltd.), 126.
16. Frankl *Anthology* 179-180
17. Frankl *Anthology* 186
18. Frankl *Anthology* 76.
19. Elizabeth Ruth Skoglund, *Bright Days, Dark Nights: With Charles Spurgeon in Triumph Over Emotional Pain* (Grand Rapids: Baker Books, 2000), 195.
20. Bell *Doctor's Guide* 123.

About the Author

A former high school teacher and school counselor, Elizabeth Ruth Skoglund, M.A., LMFT, is a Licensed Marriage and Family Therapist in private practice in Southern California. She is a certified bereavement facilitator for both adults and children. She is the author of more than 40 books and numerous magazine articles, at one time wrote a weekly newspaper column, and has appeared on many TV and radio talk shows. She has been named the Outstanding Scandinavian American 2006-2007 by the American Scandinavian Foundation of Thousand Oaks and was awarded Beautiful Activist 1973 by the Germaine Monteil Cosmetic Company and the Broadway Department Store. She has been listed in various editions of Marquis *Who's Who in America* and *Who's Who in Medicine and Health Care.*

Skoglund's books include: *Life on the Line*; *Bright Days, Dark Nights*; *Amma*; and, more recently, *Found Faithful; Divine Recycling* and *More Precious Than a Sparrow. Before I Die* and *Burnout*, as well as *Divine Recycling* and *Life on the Line*, can be found on Kindle. Skoglund's website is www.elizabethskoglund.com. She can also be found on Twitter, Facebook and LinkedIn.